Anxiety 101:
A Guide for College Students

An Anxiety Sisters E-book

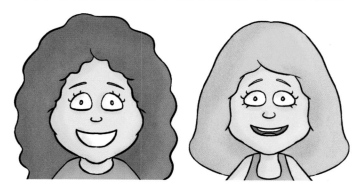

By

Abbe Greenberg, MCIS
&
Maggie Sarachek, MSW

Chapter 1

Is This Anxiety?

Yes. Probably. How do we know? Been there, done that. Also we've interviewed a lot of other people who've been there, done that. Many of us are still there, still doing that. Maybe you are too. So what does anxiety feel like? It's different for everyone, but here are some of the most common symptoms:

- Stomach distress (including nausea, puking, diarrhea, constipation, gas and cramps)
- Rapid heart beat
- Chest heaviness (hippopotamus sitting on you)
- Hyperventilating or shallow breathing (can't catch your breath)
- Dizziness (the world is spinning)
- Headaches
- Fatigue
- Shaking
- Clamminess (cold sweat)
- TBS (Tiny Bladder Syndrome—peeing constantly)
- Rashes (hives or random itching)
- Lump in the throat (difficulty swallowing)
- Skin breakouts

Really, any unpleasantness your body can produce is fair game for anxiety.

In high school, I used to go the nurse every single day with random stomach aches. Now, if it's bad, I'll just skip class and hang in my room. It's definitely not food-related. I guess it's stress. (Katie, 18)

So how can you tell the difference between being physically sick and having anxiety? It's tricky, but here are some clues: (1) symptoms are ongoing (you feel like you have the stomach flu "off and on" for an entire semester) (2) you've been to the doctor (3) you find yourself isolating or disconnecting from friends (4) you react more emotionally than is appropriate for a given situation (5) you've lost your appetite or you find yourself eating way more than usual (6) you can't fall asleep or you want to sleep all the time (7) you are crying more often and for no apparent reason (8) you are feeling overwhelmed and uneasy for no apparent reason (9) you just don't feel like yourself.

> *My first semester of college, I was crying all the time. It would come out of nowhere—there was no warning. It wasn't like something had happened. And I couldn't keep it to myself because the crying was so intense—my roommates were really worried. (Alex, 19)*

One more comment about symptoms: like bed bugs, they can relocate and multiply. In other words, your symptoms can change. Which, if you get explosive diarrhea, is a good thing.

Okay, we lied. We have another comment, and you're not going to like it. But it's the truth. If you find yourself drinking, smoking pot or using drugs to relieve your discomfort, that in itself is a huge clue that you have an anxiety issue. No judging. Like we said, been there, done that.

Chapter 2

Your Brain

We are not neurologists. In fact, we both petitioned to waive our science requirements in college. So there's that. But we have done quite a bit of research since then and feel that it is helpful to understand some brain basics. We like pictures (see above for reason)—here's the first one:

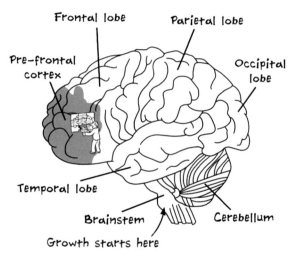

Frontal lobe

Parietal lobe

Pre-frontal cortex

Occipital lobe

Temporal lobe

Brainstem

Cerebellum

Growth starts here

Up until ten years ago, people thought that adolescent brains were just like adult brains, only smaller. Recently, neuroscientists have discovered that this is absolutely not the case. Contrary to prior beliefs, size is not the issue—it's all in the function and wiring. In fact, your brain will not be fully adult (functional and wired) until your mid-twenties!

Brains develop from back to front. This means that growth begins in the brain stem which is responsible for basic skills like breathing and swallowing. From there, the cerebellum is next, followed by the other lobes in the diagram. The last part of the brain to develop fully is the prefrontal cortex, located in the frontal lobe. The prefrontal cortex is the center of what's called executive functioning—planning, task completion, reasoning, inhibiting impulses (self-control), directing attention and problem-solving. Without this part of the brain, you would be unable to think about the future or about the consequences of your actions. You'd just be a walking sack of urges. No judgment. Been there, done that.

Figure 2 shows the brain's limbic system, including the amygdala, which is the center of emotions, and the hippocampus, which is the center of memory. In adolescent brains, the amygdala is in overdrive—it is highly sensitized and easily stimulated (thus all the high school drama). In adults, the amygdala is wired to the pre-frontal cortex so that messages can easily be transmitted between the two. So, when an adult feels, let's say, fear (a message from the amygdala), the pre-frontal cortex will assess that fear and determine a course of action based on that assessment. The pre-frontal cortex acts as a mediator between emotion and action.

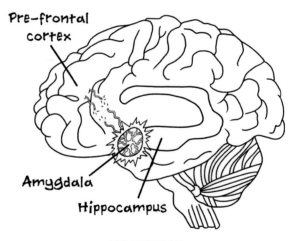

FIGURE 2

In pre-adult brains, however, the turbo-powered amygdala is not yet fully connected to the pre-frontal cortex, which means that messages will not get through as quickly or at all. Bummer, right? Well, look on the bright side: the hippocampus is also super-charged during adolescence which means your memory-making skills are way sharper than those of adults. (This is why college students are learning machines and your parents can never find their keys.)

So there is a bit of a paradox here: you have the iPhone 500 (the smartest of the smart) which has thumb-less texting (based on thoughts alone) and its own drone which delivers two am pizzas. You get the idea. The only problem is that the Wi-Fi is shitty. Which means sometimes, someone else gets your pizza.

In brainspeak, if messages aren't getting through from your amygdala to your pre-frontal cortex, there's no rational voice to control your emotions. Actions, therefore, are more impulsive and your executive function is limited. Which explains why teenagers have a reputation for impulsive, overly emotional, risky behaviors.

But that's not the end of the story. Other chemical factors influence the pre-adult brain.

- First, there's the hormone issue, but it's not what you think. The Raging Hormones Theory of Teenage Behavior is a myth. Adolescents don't actually have more hormones in their systems than do adults. The difference is that, for teenagers, the surge of sex hormones such as estrogen, progesterone and testosterone is a *new* experience for the brain. As with other new experiences (make your own analogy here), it takes time to figure out the ropes and get things right. Until then, expect mood swings.

- THP (tetrahydropregnanolone) is a steroid produced by the body in response to stress. In adults, THP quiets the nervous system. In teenagers, however, THP does just the opposite—it excites the nervous system further so it is harder to calm down.

- One more chemical to discuss: dopamine. This neurotransmitter is responsible for arousal and pleasure of all kinds—it promotes reward-seeking behavior. The release of and response to dopamine is faster and stronger in adolescents. Because the wiring in the frontal lobe is not yet fully developed, decision-making is, once again, impaired, which makes pre-adults more driven toward rewards, regardless of the risks involved.

All of these complexities leave the pre-adult brain more suscepti-ble to anxiety and depression.

The next drawing shows a map of the brain's limbic system, which is its emotional center. Of particular importance is the amygdala (which we have already discussed), often referred to as the brain's "Early Warning System," which lets the hypothalamus (the brain's "Command Center") know when it perceives that danger is near. The hypothalamus then initiates the "fight or flight" response we are so familiar with—the rapid heartbeat, the shallow breathing, the nausea, the tight muscles, the sweatiness, the dizziness, etc.

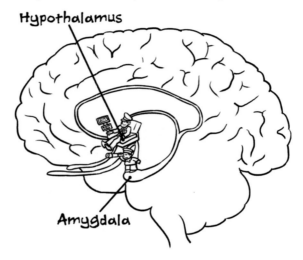

In an anxiety sufferer, the amygdala tends to overreact and send out the danger signal prematurely, too often, or too intensely, thereby sending the hypothalamus and the entire limbic system into overdrive. You may remember that the amygdala of the pre-adult is already overstimulated. So it's a double whammy. No wonder you're freaking out!

A final but really important neurological topic we need to address concerns neurotransmitters, which is a fancy name for brain chemicals. These brain chemicals transmit signals throughout the body telling, for example, the heart to beat, the lungs to breathe, and the stomach to digest. What is most important to know about these neurotransmitters is that they need to be in balance. Much like our three-tiered system of government, these guys work together and keep each other in check. (Okay, maybe not like our government.)

You may have heard of some of these neurotransmitters, of which there are several. We are going to talk about the two most well known and their connection with medication. Serotonin, most of which is found in the gut (anxious stomach anyone?), regulates mood, appetite, impulse control, sleep and libido. Norepinephrine, located in the brain, is a stimulant responsible for physiological arousal such as increased blood pressure. Clearly, these neurotransmitters have important jobs and, if unbalanced, can cause a host of problems including, but not limited to, anxiety and depression.

The medications used to treat anxiety and depression target these neurotransmitters. Selective Serotonin Reuptake Inhibitors, commonly referred to as SSRIs, are a class of medication that aims to increase deficient levels of Serotonin. (Examples of these meds include Prozac, Paxil, Zoloft, Celexa and Lexapro.) Serotonin-Norepinephrine Reuptake Inhibitors (SNRIs) are designed to target deficiencies in both Serotonin and Norepinephrine. (Examples include Effexor, Cymbalta and Pristiq.) We will talk more about these drugs and others in Chapter 6.

So let's sum things up:

1. Even though you look like an adult, your brain is not an adult brain. Not until you're about 25. The same goes for your friends.

2. Your pre-adult brain is susceptible to impulsive decision-making and difficulty with planning, evaluating consequences and completing tasks.

3. Due to the "dopamine drive," your brain craves constant stimulation and reward, and it needs more excitement than does the adult brain to feel the same gratification. For this reason, your brain is predisposed to addiction. And we're not just talking about drugs and alcohol—sex, video games, and gambling—really any activity that sets off the brain's reward center—can cause a dopamine "rush."

4. Your pre-adult brain is more prone to anxiety and depression than the adult brain.

7

What to do with all this info? Nothing in particular. It's just another way of being self-aware and understanding your strengths and possible limitations. It can also help explain behaviors that seem "out of character" or out of your control. And it should make your anxiety easier to grasp. More on this in the next chapter…

Chapter 3

Anxiety Disorders

Our experience of anxiety is rooted in the brain. As a stomach-ache is a sign of intestinal distress, so anxiety is a sign of an imbalance in the brain. In other words, anxiety is a "brain pain." Learning this changed everything for us. No longer were we to blame for our symptoms or weak for not being able to overcome them. Just like any other illness, anxiety is fundamentally a physical malfunction.

We often think of the brain as an organ in our bodies, but this is a bit of an understatement. The brain is The Organ—it controls everything from movement to emotion. Nothing in the body happens without interacting with the brain. Everyone talks about the "mind-body" connection, but this implies that each could be without the other. Which is not the case. The brain is the body and directs every bodily function. Just think of this: when you break your ankle, you lose mobility in that foot, but we do not expect this fracture to compromise your ability to SnapChat. When a part of your brain malfunctions (as in the case of a stroke), the ability to move your foot may be affected. As will possibly be your speech, your emotions, and your intellectual abilities.

So when these "brain pains" start happening more and more frequently and affect your ability to go about your day, you may be diagnosed with an anxiety disorder. The following is a list of the most commonly diagnosed anxiety disorders:

- Panic Disorder If you've experienced an anxiety attack, you would probably rather clean the bathrooms of several fraternities with a toothbrush (on a Sunday morning) than go through that again. The thing is, if you have panic disorder, you go through it often, perhaps even several times each day. As Panic Sisters, we really sympathize with these sufferers. The physical symptoms are so scary and seem to come from nowhere—one minute you're fine and the next you think you may actually die. One of the hallmarks of Panic Disorder is something we call the Anxiety Loop, which is the fear of having another anxiety attack, which can then bring on another attack. Because the panic attack experience is so hellish, understandably, sufferers avoid places they've had them. (We'll talk more about this in the next chapter.)

When I get a panic attack, I get really dizzy and spacy. I kind of zone out. My heart is beating super fast and I think I will pass out (which hasn't happened yet). It lasts about 20 minutes but it feels like forever. After, I just want to go to sleep. (Jen, 20)

- Generalized Anxiety Disorder (GAD) GAD sufferers are worriers. If you've been diagnosed with GAD, you constantly feel uneasy and often dwell on worse case scenarios surrounding everyday issues like health, relationships, schoolwork, and money. You may have difficulty concentrating (spacing out), problems sleeping, muscle tension, restlessness, irritability, and exhaustion.

I couldn't stop thinking about the paper, even after I turned it in. I was worried I hadn't done it right...I was afraid I'd blown my GPA. I kept bringing it up with my friends. They just got annoyed. They're always asking me why I can't let stuff go. The thing is, I try, but I can't stop it. I'm always worried about something. (Lin, 19)

- Social Anxiety/Social Phobia If you suffer from social anxiety, you have an extreme fear (phobia) of being judged by others in social situations and are terrified that you will humiliate yourself in front of others. Often experiencing physical symptoms of panic, Social Phobics tend to avoid social interaction such as going to parties, playing on a team, or even raising their hands in class. Social anxiety is not the same thing as shyness or introversion.

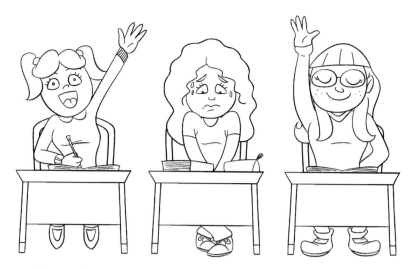

It's not like I'm antisocial or anything. It's just that I get these thoughts that I'll say something stupid or people won't like me. If I have a couple of beers, it's much easier...(Ben, 21)

- <u>Obsessive Compulsive Disorder (OCD)</u> If you have OCD, you experience uncontrollable and reoccurring anxiety-provoking thoughts (*obsessions*) and rituals or routines (*compulsions*) that you need to repeat over and over in order to relieve the anxiety caused by the obsessive thoughts. These obsessions and rituals are very intrusive and time-consuming and therefore can make the sufferer feel "stuck" or unable to move on to the next activity.

Every time I leave my apartment, I always worry that I left the stove on even though I know I didn't. I'll stand there for a while thinking about it, but I always end up going back. I have to touch each knob and say "Off." Sometimes I'll go back two or three times. (Lauren, 22)

- <u>Phobias</u> These are irrational fears that sufferers feel unable to control.

Phobic reactions are extreme and disruptive. Common phobias include spiders, elevators, clowns, thunder, vomiting, driving, flying, needles and germs, but just about anything can become a phobia. If you are phobic, you will go to great (sometimes ridiculous) lengths to avoid the object of your fear.

11

Since childhood, I have always been petrified of cockroaches—I mean, really scared. If I saw one, I would shake all over and feel sick. Once, when I was in college, I lit a chair on fire using a can of hairspray and a lighter in order to kill a roach that crawled on it. It wasn't enough to kill it—I had to completely destroy it. My roommates thought I was crazy. I had nightmares about that bug for weeks. (Abbe, 49)

- <u>Posttraumatic Stress Disorder</u> (PTSD) If you are suffering from PTSD, you have experienced or observed a trauma—like an accident, sudden death, sexual assault, violent crime, natural disaster, war or any other harmful event—from which you have been unable to recover. Depression, anxiety, and flashbacks to the incident are the hallmarks of PTSD. In addition, you may experience a state of hypervigilance (constantly being on high alert), sleep difficulties, nightmares, appetite changes, a heightened startle response, feelings of mistrust, isolation, jumpiness, crying jags, and angry outbursts. Emotional numbness and avoiding physical contact are also common with PTSD sufferers.

I was raped freshman year. It took me a long time to even say that because I thought that since I knew the guy and was in his room, maybe it was my fault. I was embarrassed to tell anyone. But I cried a lot and couldn't sleep, eat, or concentrate. My grades were terrible and I was a mess. I spent a lot of time alone in my room, and I would jump when anyone would come too near or try to hug me. This went on for months. Only after finally going to see a counselor did I realize that I was actually raped and I was suffering from PTSD. (Sophie, 21)

If any of these descriptions sound uncomfortably familiar and you haven't already, you may want to seek help. Anxiety in all its forms is treatable; don't go it alone.

Chapter 4

Anxiety Effects

If you're anxious, you are not alone. The most recent surveys of campus counseling centers revealed that anxiety has surpassed depression as the most common mental health diagnosis among college students. We are truly in the midst of an anxiety epidemic!

Speaking of depression, now's as good a time as any to talk about it. When you suffer from anxiety you feel crappy. You often don't want to even get out of bed and, certainly, not out of your dorm or apartment. Your energy is sapped, you may experience insomnia, appetite changes, and, of course, a feeling of hopelessness and despair. In other words, you display many of the symptoms of depression. Which comes first is largely a chicken-and-egg debate, but the literature in general supports a strong association between anxiety and depression (sort of like how we feel about the Kardashians—did they cause America's downfall or are they a result? Who knows, but there is clearly a correlation).

We know you already know this, but there are enormous academic consequences arising from untreated anxiety disorders. You may have difficulty concentrating, sleep problems (which then causes waking up problems), and debilitating physical symptoms. All of this leads to exhaustion and an inability to complete your work on time or at all. Even going to class, much less participating or interacting with professors during office hours, is a tall order. In other words, academic hurdles become road blocks and what is already challenging becomes insurmountable.

Perhaps one of the most insidious consequences of anxiety is what we call "Shrinking World Syndrome." In a nutshell, SWS occurs when you stop doing activities because you believe they may provoke anxiety. SWS starts quietly—you decide not to join a club or stop going to parties. Then you find yourself spending more and more time alone. Before you know it, you are reluctant to go anywhere. It feels like your world has gotten so small—that you can take only a few steps that are safe before you plunge into icy unknown waters.

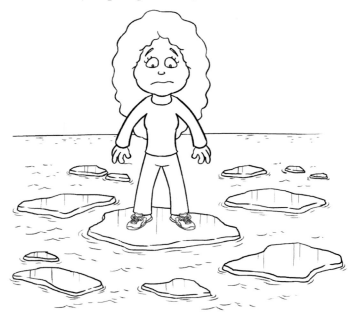

It started with a panic attack at the movies—suddenly I couldn't breathe and my heart was racing. The walls were closing in on me so I just left right in the middle. The next week, my boyfriend wanted to go see another movie. I got panicky just thinking about it. So I avoided the movies. When I got that claustrophobic feeling at a party, I stopped going to crowded places altogether. (Marisa, 25).

SWS sufferers don't retreat only from the places they feel anxious; they avoid places they think *might* make them anxious. This very quickly casts a pretty wide net. As more and more places become off limits, your room becomes the one place that feels "safe." The danger in retreat is that you believe everything will be okay if you can just get back there. What we are talking about here is not just a geographical shrinking but an emotional one as well. You convince yourself that you simply cannot handle being out in the world, and you prove it to yourself when you stay isolated.

You may be thinking that SWS is pretty extreme, but you don't have to spend all your time alone in your room to suffer from this syndrome. So don't assume you are free of SWS just because you go to class. The real issue is whether you or your anxiety decides how you spend your time.

Closely related to SWS is the feeling of isolation that anxiety causes. It's not just a physical isolation but a deep feeling of loneliness. Anxiety makes you feel out of sync with everyone else you perceive to be "normal." Not to mention how depleted you feel after spending so much energy managing your physical and emotional symptoms. You just don't have anything left to give.

I was so anxious and sad that I really couldn't think about making friends. I spent most of my time in my dorm on Instagram. All of my high school friends seemed to be having so much fun. Aside from my roommates, I did not really get to know anyone else. Going out just felt too hard. I would spend a lot of time on the phone with my parents...(Eva, 19)

Chapter 5

More Snags

Let's recap. First you have that wiring issue with the pre-adult brain. Then you have an anxiety disorder. But wait—there's more. There are other issues that contribute to this emotional soup.

- <u>High School Fallout</u> You've survived high school, but not without scars. Let's be honest—the amount of pressure you dealt with just to get into college is insane. (We never could have handled what you went through.) You arrived at college pre-loaded with stress. You're already exhausted!

- <u>Separation Anxiety</u> For many of you, college is the first time you are living away from home for any length of time. This transition is more difficult than most people think. Homesickness is only part of it. Now you are going to have to do things for yourself—things your parents may have taken care of before. We're talking everything from laundry to making appointments to managing your own schedule. And if you've been really connected with your parents, it can be very hard to be away from them.

- <u>ADHD/ADD</u> We don't need to tell you what this is, but we do need to acknowledge that difficulty focusing, planning, completing tasks and organizing is not going to make the challenges of college life any easier. Also, few people have ADD/ADHD without anxiety—they go together like ~~midterms and Adderall~~ peanut butter and jelly.

- <u>Money</u> College today is completely unaffordable; the reality is that most of you will graduate in debt after struggling for four years to pay the bills. This often means that college kids need to work long hours in addition to keeping up with schoolwork.

- <u>Social Media</u> Let's face it, your generation is plugged in 24/7. You never get a break from your phones and your various social media accounts. While certainly there are benefits to this, the flip side means more pressure—you can never be "off." Additionally, social media is hyper-stimulating, and, as we said before, the pre-adult brain is already overcharged. And then there's the comparisons that inevitably arise when everyone is posting their highlight reels, which makes it pretty hard not to develop FOMO.

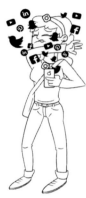

- <u>Societal Pressures</u> From the time you pass puberty through adulthood, our society permits and sometimes even encourages commentary on female body size and shape. Whether this commentary is positive or negative, it is invasive and demeaning. Culturally-sanctioned judgment only makes us feel less comfortable in our own skins.

- <u>Expectations</u> How many of you have been told that college will be the best time of your life? We're betting that most of you have heard something to that effect. Sometimes reality looks different than the expectations, and this can lead to deep disappointment, especially when all your friends are posting pictures of their fabulous college lives. First semester, for many, does not match up with what they had envisioned. Very few people meet their best friends Freshman year. And— here's the shocker—sometimes college is not the highlight of your life.

- <u>Pre-existing Conditions</u> If you struggled with either depression or anxiety in high school, you are more predisposed to struggle with it in college. The good news here is that you've already been through it and know what it is; as such, you can be prepared and set up your resources in advance.

- <u>Adults Who Don't Understand</u> We're talking about parents, professors, bosses, coaches and anyone else who calls you "lazy," "unfocused," "irresponsible," or otherwise trivializes or misconstrues your anxiety. We'd like to tell you to avoid these folks, but clearly that's impossible. So what should you do? First, remember that, for the generation before you, mental disorders carried a great stigma—people, therefore didn't openly discuss their symptoms or even that they had a disorder at all. There was too much shame. People would rather be thought of as lazy or irresponsible than anxious. Through much effort, this is starting to change. But not everyone is there yet. This means, unfortunately, that it falls on you to educate the adults in your life. You can show them written information, like this book, websites, documentaries, etc. or, if you would like some help with the explanation, you can ask a mental health counselor to intervene on your behalf. Or you can give them our email address (absandmags@anxietysisters.com) and we will happily respond.

Part of our mission as Anxiety Sisters is to eradicate, once and for all, the stigma surrounding mental health issues. We are doing this through education and by trying to bring the conversation into the mainstream. You can be part of this effort by doing the same.

Chapter 6

Treatments & Strategies

Let's start with therapy because that will probably be the first step in managing your anxiety. The most common type of therapy used to treat anxiety disorders is called Cognitive Behavioral Therapy or CBT. While there are many different types of CBT, the emphasis generally is on changing thoughts in order to alter behavior. The good news is that CBT is a short-term commitment and very focused on tangible results. Almost every college or university has a campus counseling center. That is an excellent place to start.

> *I was in such bad shape over this one Saturday that my parents told me I needed to go to the student health center or they were coming to pick me up. So I went to the health center and they checked to make sure I was okay for the weekend—that I wasn't going to hurt myself. Then they set up an appointment at the Counseling Center first thing Monday morning. The counselor I saw that Monday became my lifeline. She really helped me get through it. (Sami, 20)*

Depending on how much anxiety is interfering with your ability to function, therapy may not be [quick] enough. Medication can be an excellent tool in managing your disorder. In most cases, there are two types of meds used in anxiety treatment. The first of these are Selective Serotonin Reuptake Inhibitors (SSRIs) like Prozac, Zoloft, Lexapro, Celexa, and Paxil, to name a few. You take this type of medication every day. The good news is that these drugs are not addictive and tend to work for most people. The bad news is that SSRIs must build up in your system in order to be effective so it can take up to 6-8 weeks to get full relief (some lucky people experience relief within the first couple of weeks).

> *It took a while to work—like maybe a month. But then it really took the edge off. I could concentrate enough to do my work again. (Kayla, 21)*

The other class of drugs used to treat anxiety are Benzodiazepines. You may recognize Ativan, Valium, Xanax and Clonopin, which are all members of this group. Unlike SSRIs, these meds are taken on an "as needed" basis. They are sedatives which provide an immediate calming effect, which means they are great for treating panic. HOWEVER, these drugs can be very addictive, especially for the pre-adult brain. We don't want to sound like protective parents here, but we have to tell you the truth:

MIXING BENZOS WITH ALCOHOL OR OTHER RECREATIONAL DRUGS CAN BE FATAL.

The following are non-medical strategies that can be used to manage anxiety. Most of these are free and all can be used at any time without side effects.

- <u>TLC</u> This is our go-to strategy for acute anxiety or panic. Here's how you do it: (1) **Talking** is about saying words to yourself <u>ALOUD</u>. Those words can be anything soothing or a particular mantra you like. But you must at least whisper the words so your ears can hear them. Why? Because research has shown that your brain "listens" to what you tell it in your own voice. So what you do is repeat words or phrases over and over again in a calming tone. Our favorites include:

  "This too shall pass," "Breathe in, breathe out," "I am okay," and "Ride it out" but you can pick your own.

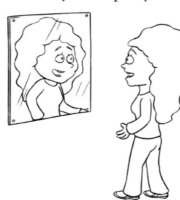

(2) **Loosening** is about freeing yourself from all constraints. It involves getting as naked as you appropriately can. Take off your [seat]belt, undo your jeans, pull out that hair clip, unclasp your bra, take off your shoes. Remove anything that makes you feel constricted. Give your belly as much room to expand as possible so you can take deeper breaths.

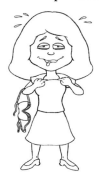

(3) **Cooling** is about bringing your body temperature down. Anxiety often makes us extremely hot (no, we mean temperature). Our fight or flight response has released all that adrenaline which serves to rev up our system (thus the rapid heartbeat, flushing, muscle tightness, and sweating). Cooling down can reset your body and cause it to stop sending out all that adrenaline, thereby allowing your heart rate to slow and your muscles to relax. Cooling involves any or all of the following: air conditioner or a fan, a cold shower or splashing cold water on your face and neck, opening windows if the air is crisp, a cool cloth on your forehead or neck, an icepack at the base of your spine, sucking on ice cubes or peppermint, or even a very cold glass of water to drink.

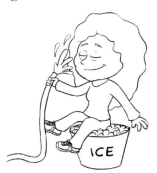

- <u>Breathing</u> Take a breath in through your nose as deeply as you can. Then release it through your mouth with a whooshing sound. This is called a calming breath—the intake of oxygen signals your brain that it needs to send out some "feel good" chemicals. Several calming breaths may be all you need to relax your stress reaction. If not, try this: Breathe in through your nose to the count of 4. Hold your breath for 4 counts. Breathe out for 4 counts. After you've got that going, repeat to the count of 5. Gradually increase the number until you are feeling better.

- <u>Grounding</u> Anxiety is a state of unreality; it results from an erroneous command from the brain to get ready to flee or fight an enemy that doesn't really exist. It's a giant screw-up. Grounding is an exercise you can do to help your brain see its error and allow your body to resume a more relaxed state. Here's how it works in 5 easy steps:

    1. Describe (talk to yourself) or write down 5 things you can see right now.
    2. Describe 4 things you can feel/touch right now.
    3. Describe 3 sounds you can hear right now.
    4. Describe 2 things you can smell right now.
    5. Describe 1 thing you can taste right now.

  By the time you finish the last step, you will have distracted yourself from the anxiety and brought yourself back into the current moment.

- <u>Bookending</u> This strategy involves creating a positive activity on either end of an anxiety-provoking event. For example, if you know that giving a presentation will cause you to feel panicky, you might "bookend" that class with something fun. It's kind of like getting a lollipop at the end of the doctor's visit—a reward for having survived the challenge. But, perhaps even more importantly, bookending involves a "lollipop" before the appointment even occurs. We say this is the more important bookend because, if you don't have one in place, more often than not, your dread will overcome you and you might decide to skip the class altogether. One great "before the event" bookend is spending time with or calling a supportive friend who can help talk you through it a bit. You can even decide to meet that same friend after the deed is done to celebrate. Or you can just do what we do—eat chocolate.

- <u>Naming</u> Visualizing your anxiety can be a great strategy to manage it. It may sound a bit juvenile, but many adult Anxiety Sisters have used this technique successfully. Here's how this works: close your eyes and try to picture what your anxiety looks like. Is it human? An animal? What color is it? Does it have teeth or claws? If you are artistic, you can even try to draw it. The next step is to name your anxiety. It sounds silly, but, if we treat our anxiety as a living thing, if we can yell at it or send it to its room, we take away its power—we regain control. Here is what Abbe's anxiety looks like (their names are Worry, Panic & Fear):

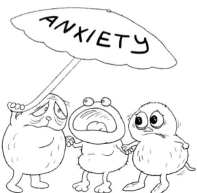

- <u>Spin Kits</u> We believe in preparing for anxiety (perhaps even more than preparing for class). We have found that having some things on hand to use during an anxiety attack can be extremely helpful in getting ourselves through the situation. Since we always think of anxiety as "spinning," we call these preparations Spin Kits. Here are a few ideas for what to include in your own Spin Kit: (1) Since our senses are often hyper-stimulated when we are anxious, anything that can soothe them might be helpful. We may have something that smells like lavender (lotion) or something with a strong taste, such as a peppermint or lemon drop. And don't just think about taste and smell. Things that soothe our senses of touch (a worry stone or soft piece of fabric) are excellent anxiety remedies too. (2) Things that distract us from our physical sensations are also great soothers. These can include music, a picture of a calming scene or a page from an adult coloring book to work on. Needlework is another great way to distract you from your anxiety symptoms. (3) Items that will help you do TLC (see above)—for example, written mantras or a cool cloth—are also helpful. (4) If they work for you, don't forget to include over-the-counter or prescription medications that alleviate uncomfortable symptoms.

- <u>Support Teams</u> One of the most powerful ways to deal with your anxiety is to make sure that you are not doing it alone. All of us, at any age, need a support team to deal with this brain illness. Whomever you can turn to for help can be part of this team. Some college students have told us that their parents and other family members are really supportive. Some students have close friends that really get it. Other people have been able to bond with a professor, religious leader, RA, coach, college advisor, or even a high school teacher. Being able to connect with a counselor (either at college or from home) and/or a psychiatrist or internist who can prescribe medication is really helpful. Just to be clear, not all counselors are created equal! If you don't feel that your counselor is helping you, please ask for someone else—you don't have to worry about hurting anyone's feelings. It's part of the job. Last but not least, let your advisor and/or professors know if you are struggling and it is affecting your work. More and more effort is being made to train faculty to understand mental health issues better. We cannot promise that they will be supportive, but it is worth giving it a try. We are always here, too, and would love to hear from you!

- <u>Soothers</u> These are items and activities that lots of Anxiety Sisters we've interviewed swear by. Some examples are lavender, Bach's Rescue Remedy (an all natural tongue spray), listening to or making music, spending time in nature, knitting and crochet, worry stones, meditation, reflexology, yoga, acupuncture, blowing bubbles (not gum, the stuff with the wand), and biofeedback.

  I knitted away my anxieties since I was 8 years old, billions of stitches... (Alene, 90)

- <u>Self-care</u> There's so much that falls into this category. Really anything that renews you and gives you joy can be self-care. And when you are dealing with an anxiety disorder, it is even more essential that you care for yourself. Self-care is not always a healthful or constructive activity (like, say, going to Pilates). It can be an ice cream cone, a Netflix binge, or treating yourself to a manicure.

- <u>Food</u> Many "experts" recommend eliminating certain types of foods in order to ease anxiety. Sugar, caffeine, gluten and dairy are usually the targets of the food police. Here's the thing. Every body is different. You need to figure out what feels right. If a double shot of Espresso doesn't seem to affect your anxiety, by all means, keep drinking it! But it might be a good idea to pay attention for a week or two, just to see if anything you are ingesting is making your anxiety worse.

- <u>Exercise</u> Everyone and their mother seems to think that a vigorous cardiovascular workout is good for managing anxiety. In fact, we're sure you've heard about the studies that show that exercise is as effective as medication in treating mental disorders. Here's our take: movement can help relieve stress. But if you have panic disorder or acute anxiety, vigorous exercise heats up the body and increases your heart rate, which mimics and may even bring on anxiety symptoms.

I was such a gym rat—I used to run on the treadmill every day for 45 minutes. But then I started to feel like crap after. Like really anxious. One of the trainers told me that heavy cardio can make you have a panic attack. I didn't believe her, but it kept happening so I finally stopped running. Now I walk and do yoga. It's much better. (Taylor, 22)

- <u>Sleep</u> This is a tough one, as college is not typically a restful time in your life. But as long as we're handing out advice, we might as well go all the way. The typical pre-adult brain requires 9 hours of sleep per night in order to perform optimally the following day. Also, lack of sleep can exacerbate anxiety symptoms. We were in college once too, so we can hear how ridiculous this sounds. But still. Try.

Chapter 7

Resources

We hate to lecture (hello, we're parents—that was an obvious lie), however we really believe it is important to find an anxiety support team (family, friends, mentors, coaches, professors, pets) and to know where and when to get help. An excellent place to start is your college counseling center, which you should explore before you need it. In other words, find out where it is located on campus and put their number in your phone for easy access. You can even stop by after you've settled into your room/apartment and see if you can meet with a counselor to help you with the transition. You'll be beating everyone else to the punch so you won't have to worry about waiting for appointments.

In a crisis—you are feeling extremely ill or are having thoughts of hurting yourself—you may want to go straight to the medical center or ER unless you are lucky enough to be at one of the schools which has a dedicated mental health emergency program. Again, this is a good thing to find out about before you get to campus.

Aside from these centers, there are a number of other resources you may wish to check out:

Anxiety Sisters (anxietysisters.com)

Ok, we know you know about us. You can reach us through our website (Contact Us), our Facebook page, through Instagram (theanxietysisters) or email us at absandmags@anxietysisters.com. We promise that, if you reach out to us, we will respond quickly.

Active Minds (activeminds.org)

This is a student-run organization with chapters on different college campuses. Like the Anxiety Sisters, this organization is aimed at ending the stigma connected with brain illness. Through peer education, they teach and encourage their fellow students to seek help. Plus, they have rockin' parties (just seeing if you are paying attention).

Anxiety and Depression Association of America or ADAA (adaa.org)

If your therapist isn't a member of this group, he/she should be. This is the largest professional organization of mental health folks (they are also open to students and people that want to learn more about mental health issues). This group is really up on all the latest research and they have an excellent website and newsletter. It is a great place to learn more about anxiety or any other mental health issues.

The JED Foundation (jedfoundation.org)

This is an organization founded by the parents of a student who committed suicide while in college. They are determined to help build "emotional safety nets" for young people by working with colleges on mental health issues. Schools who are designated "JED Campuses" have demonstrated a strong commitment to providing "comprehensive mental health programming" for their student body. They also have an active social media presence with excellent resources and an online resource called ULifeline (ulifeline.org) for immediate help and support.

National Alliance on Mental Illness (nami.org)

NAMI is a fantastic organization started and run by families living with mental illness. They do advocacy work, have support chapters just about everywhere, and are full of information of just about every type. The support aspect is really key here and it is life-changing for many people living with mental illness.

National Institute of Mental Health or NIMH (nimh.nih.gov)

This is the US government's mental health research branch so it is a great resource for statistics and to find out what scientists are up to in the mental health world.

<u>The Trevor Project</u> (thetrevorproject.org)

This organization is focused on helping to end suicide and mental health crises among LGBTQ young people. Their Trevor Lifeline is a wonderful program which connects callers with trained counselors who provide a safe, nonjudgmental environment in which to talk.

<u>Crisis Text Line</u> (crisistextline.org)

We know the founding supervisor for this group, and she is the most dedicated, caring soul. Her organization provides free, 24/7 support for anyone in crisis. Just text 741741 from anywhere in the USA to be connected with a trained Crisis Counselor and let your fingers do the talking.

One particularly effective way of coping with any disorder is by connecting with others who are in the same boat. We started the Anxiety Sisterhood for this very reason—we wanted to provide a safe, nonjudgmental community where we could share stories, strategies, complaints, experiences and laughter. Just interviewing fellow sufferers and writing about our collective experiences has been such an important component of our recoveries. In fact, the more anxiety sisters we talk to, the easier we find managing our own anxiety. We envision anxiety sisters from all over the world reaching out and helping fellow sufferers get on their feet…this is our mission.

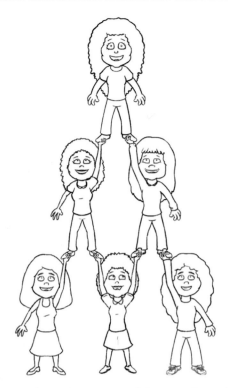

Creating the Sisterhood has been our lifeline, and we'd like to invite you to be part of it. Please visit our free website at http://anxietysisters.com and join our rapidly growing sisterhood (brothers are welcome too!). Just being part of the conversation can make a difference for you and for so many others who are struggling to manage anxiety in all its forms.

Made in the
USA
Middletown, DE